ENCLOSURES

ENCLOSURES

reflections from the prison cell
and the hospital bed

poetry by Shirin Karimi

cover design by Liz Calka

text design by Sonia Tabriz

BleakHouse Publishing

2011

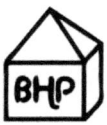

BleakHouse Publishing
NEC Box 67
New England College
Henniker, New Hampshire 03242
www.BleakHousePublishing.com

Robert Johnson - Editor
Sonia Tabriz - Managing Editor
Liz Calka - Art Director

Susan Nagelsen - Senior Consulting Editor
Erin George, Charles Huckelbury, Shirin Karimi, Chris Miller,
& Saba Tabriz - Consulting Editors
Carla Mavaddat - Assistant Art Director

Copyright © 2011 by Shirin Karimi

All rights reserved. No part of this book shall be reproduced or transmitted in any form or by any means, electronic, mechanical, magnetic, photographic, including photocopying, recording or by any information storage and retrieval system, without prior written permission of the publisher. No patent liability is assumed with respect to the use of the information contained herein. Although every precaution has been taken in the preparation of this book, the publisher and author assume no responsibility for errors or omissions. Neither is any liability assumed for damages resulting from the use of the information contained herein.

ISBN-13: 978-0-9797065-7-8
ISBN-10: 0-9797065-7-2

Printed in the United States of America

For my parents,

Who taught me to write and to dream.

CONTENTS

Acknowledgments

Skin - 1

Seedlings - 3

Dancer - 5

Smothered - 7

Dirty Fingers, Dirty Body - 9

A Proclamation, A Blessing - 11

My Feminine Charms - 13

No Longer Human - 15

Crazies - 17

Monologue: Inspired By Kerry Max Cook - 19

Just Breathe - 21

Aborted Youth - 23

Scholarly Pursuit - 25

Binding Factors - 27

Lost, Never Found - 29

Eve's Apples - 31

Most Likely To Be A Socialite - 33

3 Months - 35

Will You Accept This Call? - 37

The Glass Coffin - 39

Try To Talk - 43

Weight Training - 47

My Terrorist - 49

My Intimates - 51

License To Kill - 53

A Master At His Craft - 55

A 10-Year-Old's Wish - 57

To Love And To Be Loved - 59

Weightless - 63

A Perfect Way To Start The Day - 65

The Orchestra - 67

Anxiously Awaited - 69

The Stairs That Stare - 71

About the Author

About the Designers

ACKNOWLEDGMENTS

I am deeply grateful to American University for giving me the opportunity to pursue so many wonderful interests during my four years here. I could not ask for a better college experience and will remember the lessons and the friendships for the rest of my life.

I thank all of my professors who have contributed so much to my education and shared their passion for their special fields. I am especially indebted to Professor Robert Johnson, a most supportive mentor who enlightens all his students with deep knowledge and compassion for those relegated to the forgotten corners and hidden institutions of our society. From introducing me to the criminal justice system in an elective two years ago to his unending encouragement for the production of this book, he serves as an example on the wonder of teaching to all who know him.

After taking Professor Johnson's classes, I began noticing similarities between the prison world and the medical field that I am pursuing. In drastically different settings, there is one uniting similarity: the perseverance of the spirit beyond the confining walls. Thus, these poems would not have been written without the inspiration drawn from the people in the justice and medical systems. In particular, I am grateful to Yale New-Haven Hospital and Georgetown University Hospital for allowing me to work among so many people who teach me the value of life and faith. I also thank the countless unnamed prisoners whose own creative works have moved me to learn more about their triumphs and setbacks in an unfamiliar world.

SKIN

His skin is unblemished
So I don't quite believe him when he says he has skin cancer.
But why would he joke about that?

His skin is untarnished.
In fact, it glows, unfailingly, reflecting his joy and his youth
Even if underneath, he is sick.

His skin has some freckles. Innocent sprinklings from the sun.
Beauty marks for some, they are painted on his soft flesh
Almost deliberately around his collarbone,
Framing his strong shoulders.
Hard to believe those dots hide
Something monstrous underneath.

I can't see what lies beneath. Do I even want to imagine it?
He is perfection on the outside.

SEEDLINGS

I can see her garden.
Little seedlings
Sprouting from the shimmering surface of her head.

They are tiny,
So wispy
One breeze could carry them far away
And she would be left with nothing again.

But no malicious wind, no malignant character dare touch her.
For beneath those gentle seedlings
Lies the strong, fertile soil,
A breeding ground that anchors the seeds deep
Never resigning, never relaxing its grip.

The soil is she
Resilience herself.

DANCER

Her passion: dancing.
I can see that love flare in chestnut eyes
Unadorned by eyelashes.
I can picture her in a mirrored studio,
Her soft body undulating like gentle waves,
Circulating, rotating in a come-hither dance.
I can imagine her throwing her head back in ecstasy
As she masters the moves,
A prima dancer before a mesmerized audience.
But when I ask her how the dancing is going now,
There are only ashes instead of burning fire.
Her shoulders sag, burdened by the invisible load of gravity
That holds her in place, motionless.
She seemed strong. Still.
But it wasn't a matter of strength.
For that glittering outfit would not cover her port*
And would unmask her true identity
Even if the only identity she knows is dancer.

*Note: The implantable port allows for cancer treatments and blood transfusions without repeated needle sticks. It is inserted into a vein in the chest.

SMOTHERED

I'm trapped in this infernal cave.
Light no longer exists
And I think time too has disappeared with the light.
Not even a sliver of anything to hold on to.
I am mired in this quagmire,
Slowly sinking,
Inevitable death approaching.

I can hear the Boatman come, his oars softly breaking the water.
I can't tell his exact arrival, but he comes.
I wish that he would take me quick, without pause
So I may be delivered without pain
But that is not how the world operates today
And thus I am doomed.
I am young but I feel as though I am merely biding my time
Counting every grain of life to reassure myself of life's existence
That life will continue when I'm gone
Since I know I will disappear into the mist soon.

But wait! I can see something beyond the cave.
It is small but it is there.
And suddenly, I am free from these terrible sweats,
These aching pains.

Where before I couldn't swallow, now my greedy mouth engulfs
Precious air

And I am free from this captivity.
Free from the prison of my body.

DIRTY FINGERS, DIRTY BODY

They are coming.
All 10 of them.
They look innocent enough
In their puffy, padded outfits
But looks can be deceiving.

One of them points to me,
The talon accusatory and sharp,
The eagle spotting its meal.
It crooks upwards, harsh, full of force.
They are coming.

They are coming.
Now.

I shuffle towards them.
Knowing what is to come.
Knowing what they are going to do to me.

They've gotten hold of me.
Pincers.
5 at the right leg,
5 at the left.
Working their way up.

So

Slowly.

Tantalizing.

Like the way I used to give my wife a massage after work.

That way

They can't go too fast.

It delays my deliverance.

A PROCLAMATION, A BLESSING

They've given me a cot
So hard I can feel my spinal cord
Tangled like a jump rope when I wake up.

They've given me a place to shit.
My Liberty to do my business
Confined by the termite-ridden cover
My Freedom to move limited by the bleak Arctic of the cell.

I thank them.

By imprisoning my body,
They've broken the shackles of my mind.

No longer a slave to deprivation
Waiting for the opening of the pearly gates to open my cell door.

I am free and they have bestowed freedom upon me
Pride: a foreign concept, a fleeting wisp of an idea
Now I can feel it coursing through my cracked-up veins
A feeling I have never known
For it used to be a sin to be proud, to feel pride in a killer.

I am reborn.

I am the phoenix slowly rising from burnt ashes.

My beauty will blossom, my potential will grow

As I give the gift of knowledge to my brothers

As my brothers have given the priceless pearl to me.

They can steal my cigarettes

They will never steal this from me.

MY FEMININE CHARMS

Don't be fooled by my pretty face.
These lips that you long to kiss,
Two plump, shimmering portals of ecstasy,
They hide fangs that will lovingly trace my affection for you
Before sinking the glistening ivory into your bruised skin.

My body,
A temple that pilgrims have journeyed to worship before,
It holds holy relics, mystical, magical,
Rivaling those of Bethlehem.
These arms that wrap around your curves
Enhanced by the nine months that you have borne the lofty title,
Mother Goddess,
They embrace your body, O Venus, before slowly
Rising to your chest,
Your shoulders,
Your neck of grace that I compress like pottery clay.

My nails, long ovals of reflecting rose and white crescent,
They slice through skin with the ease of a kitchen knife,
Leaving my mark of artistry behind.
Beauty is the most effective disguise.

NO LONGER HUMAN

They call me monster now.
I don't understand.
I have a face, a fully functional body,
A heartbeat.
When you touch me, my body reacts to the stimulus.
Is it really my fault I sneer instead of smile?
Gnaw instead of eat?
Am I so repulsive because I enjoy using my God-given muscles
To wield an axe instead of shaking your hand?
No, I am human.
Merely the hidden facet of humanity
That is covered in mud in a diamond mine.

CRAZIES

Let me introduce to you my friends,
Me, myself, and I.

They never leave
Even when I ask them to
Even when I grab them and try to force them out.

They remain.
Stubborn and unforgiving.

They take on different voices too
And are pretty good at it,
So I pretend that I'm watching a sitcom
But the director never calls "cut"
And I can't tell one scene from the next.

I tell them to shut up
If only for a minute, if only for a second.

My efforts are in vain
For my friends are deaf to everything outside themselves.

But no matter how much I complain,
I should be grateful.

Most people don't have a single friend.
Look at me, I have three.

MONOLOGUE
INSPIRED BY KERRY MAX COOK

When I was young and naïve,
I got a tattoo of a skull on my bicep one night in Tijuana.
I hid it from my parents, showed it off to my friends.

Now I have another tat,
That can never be hid, will never be showed off.
It stares at me with fiendish eyes when
I look at myself in the mirror.
Sneers at me when I make love to my wife.
I am Dante and it is Lucifer
But I am forever trapped in Hell
Unable to escape into the next world.

I try to pretend
It's written in a different language
Since good pussy doesn't sound very appealing in English.*
Maybe it means strong warrior or faith heals all,
Some crap like that.

I have a secret to confess.
When I'm in the shower,
(and I know this is stupid)
I try really hard to scrub it off
I take my wife's loofah and just go to work on the fucking brand

Until the water gets cold
And my wife yells at me that she needs the bathroom.
Maybe one day it will fade.
I hope.

---

*Note: This phrase was carved into Kerry Max Cook's body in a terrible assault while he was incarcerated on death row. He was later exonerated.

JUST BREATHE

He was my first love. I loved my husband (for a brief period of time, before the good-for-nothing jackass left us), but he was my first love. From the minute I saw him, he was up there with the good Lord in my eyes. Angel. I knew I would never feel love like this ever again. He would have my heart, always and forever. They've injected the first 2 chemicals, one to anesthetize, one to stop his breathing. When he was born, he stopped breathing for a few seconds. I stopped breathing for 10.

The last injection went in. His cobalt eyes were closed and I thought about how I had memorized his every orbit of blue that communicated his fears, his hopes, his failing faith. I tried to see if his body responded in any different way but it didn't. Maybe there was an imperceptible shudder when his soul left his body. I hoped he was at peace. No longer breathing but all that I could hope for was eternal peace, his deprived peace for so, so long.

I could feel my breath as my diaphragm rose and fell, I could pace it through the routines I learned from 20 years of yoga. Fresh oxygen in, carbon dioxide out, a procedure my body has learned and excelled at without fail. But now, he is not breathing. And I don't want to anymore.

> Can I hold my breath forever, until I finally expire?
> I think I can, maybe if I succeed,

God will give me what I want.
So I try, I suck in my last breath,
Sharply, like a sudden injection,
My ruddy cheeks puff out to enclose the
Precious molecules
They are taking him away now
My last chance
But I still have breath left in me and
It is not running out fast enough
My chest heaves, I feel woozy

And I finally succumb and let the relieving air
Flood my ravaged body
He is gone.
And I have just missed him.
But I'll keep trying to see him again
Life is not life without him
And I stopped breathing when he did.

ABORTED YOUTH

"Grandpa Eugene, tell me a story. Tell me about when you were young."

"My child, I was just like you. You know how your momma and daddy tell you that you are like a bright star, you can light up anything you're so talented? Well, you get that from me, Charlie. I was the smartest kid in elementary school. Can you believe it, I used to pay people to do their math homework for them? The other kids, they would beg to get me as their lab partner or presentation buddy. I loved the attention. Always wanted to be in the spotlight, since Larry would beat me at everything. Me and Larry, we would wrestle on Momma and Daddy's bed and he would always beat me, but I kept thinkin', one day, I'm gonna beat him, I'm gonna be stronger. But anyway, I loved to build model airplanes and I would hang them from my room and Larry knew the way to get under my skin was to take the airplanes down from the ceiling and scatter them all over the trailer. I wanted to grow up and build real planes. Well, when I was 13, I really wished I could build them airplanes, maybe one of them would be big enough to fly me out of that cell. But they didn't let me have no materials, you know 'cause of them razor blades and hot glue, they thought I might attack my cellie or those jumpy guards or sumtin'. But Charlie, you're too young to hear about crazy things like this. I was too young to be in that cell. All I wanted was to go and wrestle Larry again but he just became stronger and taller and I'm like this now. Well, I haven't seen Larry since I came here but your momma and daddy are awful nice to let you come in here and see me. I'm the only one whose grandbaby visits, did you know that? Oh Charlie, they're ringing the bell now, we have to say good-bye. But that's ok, honestly, I don't know what else to tell you. I stopped being young a long long time ago, I don't really remember what being young was. Just airplanes and Larry and those don't exist anymore. Just give me a kiss baby. Bye Charlie, I'll see you in three months.

SCHOLARLY PURSUIT

I thought by coming to prison,
I could finally work on my-
No, scratch that, I didn't know what I would work on,
I just thought I would get the chance
To work on something!
Maybe I would be the next great American novelist,
Someone Updike or McCarthy
Would write to in admiration:
"Dear Isaac Deepwater, Convicted Felon, your frank and
Stirring usage of Metafiction has …"
Some fawning b.s. that I could feed on for days and days
Instead of the disgusting porridge for breakfast.
Ok, so if not a novel, a memoir!
My reflections on life with a coke-addled whore of a
Mother who would bring me along
For the sick old guys to "play" with.
That would be a bestseller, right?
So if that heartbreaking subject is too intense for the
General population, how about stream-of-consciousness
Narratives from a prisoner's perspective?
Hmmmm, that could work, let's try it….
"Cocksucka, I'mma cut you next time I see you!"

"You shut the fuck up or you and this wand are gonna be
Getting real friendly with each other!"

Oh God, how do you expect me to-
"Did you see that, Guard, Williams tried to shank me!"
How can I write like-
"You best be getting me my money
Or yo arm will be the ashtray
For those new cigarettes I got yo ass."
How can I write like this?
I'm trying my best here but the noise never stops.
It NEVER STOPS.

Ugly words keep circling in my brain so I am in constant
Pursuit of the appropriate adjective, the right metaphor,
That perfect dialogue
Between the protagonist and the enemy.
Clinking, clamoring, jumbling noise.
Dissonance in my ears
Leading to dissonance in my words.

BINDING FACTORS

I was saving this for that bitch cellie,
I keep thinking that she is
Gonna jump me in my sleep,
And it is definitely not worth
Getting caught by Officer Rodriguez again
But this is a good reason,
Worth everything.
My tongue slips out of my mouth, a slithering serpent
Emerging from the hole
And takes with it the tiny blade, the sharp part worn
Down by decades of use among these classy ladies
Cellie's asleep and the guards are paying attention to
Romaro and Ellengs, four cells down.
The time is right.
Now.
I slide up my sleeve a little bit and my ghostly skin
Startles me
I haven't paid this much attention to my body
For a long time. Since they told me.
Now it's just a shell, the life has left, my heart beats
Mechanically but with no purpose.
But, I can feel the pulsations speed up a little, in
Anticipation of what I am going to do.
There it is, the branching fork of four blue veins, an inch
Down from my palm.

They beckon to me like road signs,
Directing me where to go.
It takes a couple of tries for the blade to cut through skin
But once I pierce through,
The veins are weak and submissive.
How many different shades of red can I detect in this
Palate upon my skin?
Ha, Rodriguez is noticing something's up,
Took her long enough,

I mean, hello, I'm on the ground here, redness covering
My body like a viscous blanket.
They are definitely going to take me to the hospital, I've
Lost too much blood.
And then I will see her again, two days was too short.
Baby.

LOST, NEVER FOUND

The cell is 4 by 6, tiny by any standards
Except an ant hole,
And I'm pretty sure that the ants have it better than us.
At least their tiny legs can take them anywhere,
Not confined to a caged rec area for exercise.
But the thing I'm looking for is as hopeless as trying to
Find one specific ant in the colony.
I've scoured every damn inch of this cell, thousands of
Times, over and over again.
I mean, what else can I do, I've got nothing but time.
This ant is not like the others.
The others make their presence known.
They leave little trails, microscopic prints upon the dirt.
If you look closely, you will find them.
Persistence is the key.
Dedication to the cause is the solution.
But this little ant, it takes more than those two factors.
I don't know what else to do but keep searching the same
Cracks in the cement over and over again.
Whatever I need, it eludes me.
And I'm not the only one, no.
Everybody else is looking for it too.
Funny, we all have the same name for this ant.
If we ever find it, we can look it straight in the face,
And finally….satisfaction.
We call it Justice.

EVE'S APPLES

Well, Blanca and I never really got along so they brought in a new cellie. I want to start off on the right foot this time, so I'll try and think of her as a college roommate. Something I never had. I'll be nice and patient. Maybe she'll be nice too, maybe she won't be the shankin' type. I've had enough of those, thank you very much.

I'm a little nervous, I mean, what if she doesn't like me? What if she's an addict and gets me to start doing stuff with her? Shit, my counselor would be real disappointed after a whole year. Well, I shouldn't scare myself, they're opening the door, I'll just extend my hand and welcome her to her home.

Fiona. That's her name. Fiona. Pretty name. Much better than Eve. She's a new fish, she's delicate but not brittle like the others. Her hair is clean and falls to her shoulders in waves, like in *The Birth of Venus*, that was a pretty painting in the book. And she says hello to me, not in a growl, not in a timid mutter, but in a musical rhapsody that I haven't heard for 20 years. Wow, she is young, probably 18 or 19. She looks like an athlete too, not one of those lumbering gorillas on the rugby team, but maybe a gymnast or a ballerina. The way she moves endows the tiny cell with something I've never seen before. I think they call it Grace.

I can't really see the rest of the body on account of her saggy uniform. But the uniform has been recently laundered so it actually looks good on her. She has one of those hourglass figures, I bet. I always liked those, run your hands on those curves like an undulating wave in the ocean, up and down, enjoy the ride. My body? Pathetic after three bastards and a shit-ton of crack. I don't think I am anything to be admired, but her...

Maybe we'll get real close like best friends. Dare I say, girlfriends? I'll start by giving her an innocent hug after she starts to trusting me. And then...I'll start to linger a little more on the hugs, my hands resting on her toned shoulders, drifting to that collarbone. It'll take time to pick the apples though, can't rush the apple picking season. But once it happens, I know I'll never taste anything as sweet.

MOST LIKELY TO BE A SOCIALITE

That was my proudest achievement.
Oh boy,
You have no idea how hard I campaigned for that.
There wasn't a party I didn't attend,
A keg stand I didn't do,
A football game that didn't feature my high splits on the
Field with all the hot players looking at my spanks.
I was present. Everywhere. Everytime.
You could count on me.
My poor parents, every month,
They faced a $500 cell phone bill
But luckily, I was the most popular babysitter
So I gladly paid them back.
People called me a breath of fresh air
Sweeping into the room.
All conversation stopped, all eyes were on me.
I had IT, magnetism, charisma. I was the scene.
It's weird now, not having anybody to talk to.
Except you, I mean, and you are a really good listener.
People said I was always the best listener too
But I was never a gossip like Becky was, I had values.

It used to be so noisy in the main block,
I pretended the noise was music

And I would rock out to my own private dance party
Impressing all the guys (or girls, I should say)
With my sizzling moves.
But there's no more noise, no more dancing.
I can hear music in my head so I guess that works.
It's getting louder now, my favorite song!!
Do you want to dance? No? Really,
Don't be embarrassed, it's just you and me.
We'll have a great time. No? Ok, you don't mind if I
Dance, do you? I just can't help myself. It's in my nature.

3 MONTHS

I don't mean to disgust you, but I don't think the truth should disgust anybody. Just bear with me through all of this clinical nonsense. Two weeks ago, I felt something in my groin. It was inflamed I guess, but from what? I mean, I stopped fucking guys after Andy got HIV, so how could my groin be getting any action? So I went to the infirmary. Luckily Mary, that hot nurse wasn't there so I wouldn't feel embarrassed about showing her my manly parts. Dr. Williams was real professional and gentle, he wasn't repulsed by the smells or my fraying underwear. He just palpated (I think that's the word) my groin slowly and then said I needed an X-ray. So I went and got an X-ray, pretending that I was being abducted by aliens who wanted my groin, that kept me entertained for an hour. Childish I know, but funny as hell. Take me to your leader, that sort of thing.

Dr. Williams didn't share my smile when I came back. "Ricky, you have Stage IV prostate cancer. At this rate, I would estimate you have three months to get your affairs in order." Those are the only things I remember from the conversation, I pretty much blocked the rest out. I nodded, mute, and went back to my cell since there was nothing more he could do for me. They weren't going to send me to the hospital for treatment since it was Stage IV and I wasn't feeling no pain. Yet. They said they would make me comfortable when the time came.

That confused me a lot. I never thought time would "come" again, time must roll along on its tracks, no end in sight. But now, I'm given a time. 3 months. I stopped counting months years ago. First the days went, then the months, finally the years. I mean, what good is counting time when you've got life on your hands?

I can feel a smile coming on, the sensation is unfamiliar to me and my muscles are cramped from the effort. Three months… Now I can start counting the seconds and days again. Something to look forward to. My exit date. A one way ticket out of this inferno, no looking back. So, they said God doesn't exist in this hellhole? They were wrong.

WILL YOU ACCEPT THIS CALL?

I recognize her
The same vacuous voice, devoid of meaning,
Devoid of life
Saying the same words that I hear once a week,
Every week
I recognize her.
But I wish I didn't.

There is always the slight delay
Leaving me anticipating who is on the other line.
Perhaps it is an overseas call from a traveling friend.
Or maybe an annoying telemarketer I will try to avoid.
Maybe it is simply a bad connection.
But then she starts speaking.
My excitement at its denouement.

Will you accept this call from…
She doesn't need to say Allie's name
I already know
After all, I don't have any other children in prison.

An involuntary tremor tangles the phone cord.
My husband now knows it's his Allie waiting to talk.

Should I accept it?
Should I accept her?
We're connected
Yet so far apart.

THE GLASS COFFIN

They told me I could visit Mommy today so I didn't complain when Aunt Laurie pulled the poofy polka-dot dress over my shoulders, even though she knows I hate dresses. "You want to look nice for Mommy don't you?" I scowled at her and put my shiny Mary-Janes on instead of my flip flops. It took a long time to get to Mommy. I ended up falling asleep in the car with the animal cracker crumbs leaping in the air from my dress every time Aunt Laurie went over a pothole. There were a lot of potholes in this part of Virginia.

We finally arrived and I tried to say hello to the big men who never smiled. I thought that if I was nice to them, maybe they would let me spend more time with Mommy. It never worked. One mean man stopped me and Aunt Laurie from going inside. "She can't go in with that dress Ma'am," he said in the same voice Aunt Laurie uses when I spill my glass of milk all over her furniture. "Excuse me Officer?" "It is against policy for guests to wear sleeveless attire."

Grownup talk. I ignored it and tapped my shoes against the hard concrete floor, waiting to see her like a good little girl. Aunt Laurie knelt down to talk to me. She never does that.

"Sweetie, we have to go back to the car and change out of your pretty dress, ok? Let's go put on something more comfortable for you." Yes! The dress was really starting to itch.

When the mean man saw me with my jeans and long-sleeved flannel shirt, he finally nodded to some invisible person who opened the big heavy doors for us. "Go up to that glass window and see Mommy!" Aunt Laurie exclaimed.

Glass window? I didn't understand what my aunt was talking about. Mommy did always say Aunt Laurie was the silly sister. But I went up to the high window and Aunt Laurie pulled me onto the high chair.

I didn't see Mommy. There was someone who looked like Mommy, kind of. She had the same color hair but now there was a lot less hair. I used to play with Mommy's long black curls and would beg her to tell me the story of Rapunzel. Mommy was Rapunzel, but no one could rescue this person behind the glass since she didn't have enough hair. It wasn't as black anymore either. Lots of gray. I thought only Grandma and Grandpa had gray hair.

And there was something wrong with her eyes. Everyone said you could hear Mommy's laugh by looking in her eyes. Green like Slytherin in Harry Potter. I don't have green eyes. No one else I know has emerald green eyes except for Mommy. So why did her eyes look like the color of dead grass?

The person behind the glass motioned for me to kiss her. She looked so sad that I leaned forward and puckered my lips and expected to feel a soft cheek against my mouth. All I felt was cold glass. I couldn't kiss this person. This person didn't exist. Maybe she never existed.

I wasn't having fun and I wasn't spending time with Mommy so I got up to leave without saying goodbye. Aunt Laurie stopped me and said, "Go and say bye to your Mommy." I shook my head. Mommy wasn't there. I think God took her the day they took her away from us. I haven't seen her since.

TRY TO TALK

I tried to do my assignment at the correctional facility: "Interview an inmate." Three simple words, one impossible task. First, I called the public relations officer for visiting hours. Their response: "We don't have the authority to grant you permission. You must contact the Warden's secretary." So then, I tried that number. After an hour listening to droning beeps while the automatic voice kept me on hold, I finally spoke to a secretary in his office. Some answer: "Sorry, we can't allow a visitor with no relation to the inmates." "Well, what if I want the experience to learn from him?" "No."

So, what is it they always say? If you can't get an answer, go straight to the big dog. Instead of swallowing my pride, I gulped down my fear and dialed the Warden's number. His reputation precedes him. He gave ME hell. I don't even know what he does to the poor inmates. But my professor had used his considerable influence and the Warden finally grunted his approval. Tuesday at 1. I would have 30 minutes. Better get some questions together.

The day came. I dressed in a suit (who was I trying to impress anyway?) and went through Security, pretending I was boarding a plane. Destination: Inmate A4905.

Hi. I'm Mike. What's your name?

Michael Gabriel Valley.

Good name. So what did you do to land here?

Well, I don't think stealing food to feed my baby and my pregnant wife should land anyone in the joint. But it did.

Huh.

Yeah. So how old are you?

19. How about you?

I was 19 when I got here three years ago. You must be in college. Whaddya studying?

Well, I'm undecided.

As am I.

My parents are kinda on my case. Everyone else has picked a major and everything.

Well, you can't rush these things. You deserve to find something you love. I really loved painting airplanes. That's what all these tats are.

You did those yourself?

Yeah. No planes to paint here so I did them with some ink I got from the print shop.

Whoa. Well, I'm thinking graphic design but you know what they say.

What do they say?

No money in it. My dad's pushing Econ for me. Like I could seriously study regression graphs for the next four years.

Yeah I hated Econ in high school. That's why I started working at the coffee shop. Then they laid me off when the crunch happened. Guess some Econ would have helped us all out.

So what did you do then?

I temped for a while but all the unemployed college kids wanted the jobs. Bastards didn't have a family either. I really didn't have anything.

When did you get married?

When I was 18. She made me a better person so I knew I didn't want anyone else in my life. She got pregnant right after we married. No money for the Pill, you know? And now she's four months pregnant and she and Cody are always hungry. So I pulled into a Safeway to ask for a job. Big surprise, they didn't have any. Cody was crying and Mandy was clutching her stomach. I grabbed some Ramen and milk. They grabbed me and here we are.

Jesus Christ man. They can do that?

More than you know. Funny isn't it? You can beat some jerk up in a bar and not get locked up, but steal $10 worth of groceries and you do hard time.

Dude, that's crazy. My parents pay my housing and dining bill at the beginning of the semester and I don't think twice. I'm just trying to find a date for the formal.

No girls for a handsome guy like you? That's hard to believe.

Believe it. I guess girls don't like nice guys.

I was a nice guy and I got Mandy.

You *were* a nice guy? Not anymore?

You get here and you make a choice. Stay nice or stay alive. And people don't go back to being nice. I stole groceries; they stole my heart.

WEIGHT TRAINING

I was a scrawny lad with tailored Brooks Brothers suits
To camouflage my lanky arms, my gangly legs.
Didn't have time to work out in the morning
Before the markets opened.
Now the only market I need to know is the snack market.
And I've turned to disciplining my body instead.
So where before I had a MENSA mind,
I now have enviable biceps brachii,
Pumped to perfection.

MY TERRORIST

These evil people have placed a bomb
That sits with me in my room.
It wasn't enough to merely enclose me here
As if I were a rabid dog.
No. They feel the need to place an ever-present reminder
Of death that mocks me with every tick.
Whoever designed this torture
Knew exactly what he was doing.
The ticks mimic the beat of my heart.

MY INTIMATES

The word itself shows how it holds someone in the
Closest embrace.
The first syllable. In. Not out.
Then, the middle part. Lodged safely in between.
And finally…mates.
Very appropriate.
I expected my future mate to be the first to explore with
Gentle caresses.
And now I must settle for brutes with rough hands and
Even rougher words.

LICENSE TO KILL

My brother and I loved James Bond.
LOVED James Bond.
I would be Bond and he would be the evil despot.
He's now a professor.
Bond however became depressed after the war.
Couldn't hold down a job after seeing so much death.
I ask you, how could I go on
Using my hands and my mind to further my life?
To meet someone and marry her,
To create life
When so much life was torn apart by unseen hands in front of
My innocent eyes?
I hope you understand.
My license to kill could finally be put to good use.

A MASTER AT HIS CRAFT

They say that your soul mate is a sculptor who takes a marble You and carefully uses their skill to create a more perfect work of art. Chip away at your flaws, reveal your beauty underneath. Improvement, enhancement, make you the best, better than you thought you could be. He was my Michelangelo and I was his Pieta. A block of marble converted into the holy Mary. Only he could do that to me.

But they took him away from our townhouse on Park Avenue. The family business went to that tank of sharks, the Board of Trustees, who jumped on my husband's life work as if there were blood in the water.

We bought the townhouse together in the 80's for a few hundred grand. Watched it grow into 3 million. Collected De Kooning and Chagall together at Sotheby's. Donated to Carnegie Hall. Made a life together.

Now the townhouse is a shack. There used to be joy in every antique we sought together, every Persian rug we imported, every crack in the original tile. Now, I see despair as if the cracks are broken smiles that sneer at me all day, every day.

Michelangelo. The sculptors back then used wax to cover any mistakes in their artistry. So did Jacob. Instead of using wax, he used the investors' money. Turned the most pure family business into something counterfeit.

And now, I think our marriage was the same. It looked like the finest marble, without wax, sin cera, sincere and true. But my Michelangelo was simply a master at his craft and used his wax to the best effect. The Feds have scrubbed away at the wax. All that is left are the cracks.

A 10 YEAR OLD'S WISH

AML
I can't pronounce the real thing so I stick to AML.
It's a new phrase I've had to learn.
It's not exciting like LOTR.
It's not cool like GW, the college my sister goes to.
It's just ugly and weird and unwanted.
The doctors talk about antibodies
My would-be protectors.
I just don't understand it
So I'm going to go to my room and
Bury myself in my new Lego fortress
The set that Mom bought me after the spinal tap
Hopefully the people living there will be protected by the
Plastic walls.

*Note: AML stands for acute myeloid leukemia

TO LOVE AND BE LOVED

God put love in my heart.
He put it in yours too.
And for so long, like any other,
I have longed to love and to be loved,
To hold and be held,
To find the mirror image of my soul in another
Two compliments combining to form a perfect union
More pure and true than the individual parts.
I know that my parents have done this
And their parents as well
And the thousands and thousands of nameless faces
Who came before and who will come after
As two notes, octaves apart,
Combining to form a chord of perfection
Revealing God's love to all those who will
Let their ears receive His glorious sounds.
25 years, I have been deaf to the music
But now the orchestra resounds, the timpani like
Agamemnon's advancing army
With the gentle flute's overtures, a mother's sweet caress
Delicate and forceful, powerful and tender
The vibrations from each reverberating
In the chambers of my heart.
I feel after 25 years
That I am just learning how to live

For life was not life, could not be called life
Merely a gray and tattered replica
Of what life is meant to be,
Before we met.

When before I lived only for myself
A selfish Epicurean
I now surrender solely to us.
I cannot call my heart or my mind my own
Nor my eyes nor my fingers nor my lips.
All these things and more belong to us.
I thought that I was cursed
To traverse the thorny paths of life
With my eyes focused on the ground to avoid danger
And now we can brave the forbidden world together
With eyes looking beyond the dark canopy of trees
Toward the radiance of the sun's light and glory above.

I never thought though that a barrier would be placed
Strong and sturdy
Iron and sweat
Drizzled with droplets of congealed blood
Red tears painting the ugly façade's cheeks.
As much as we try, as great as we struggle
We cannot pass
And I am once again trapped in the forest
Vulnerable to menace,
My eyes locked on the muddy sediment.

All I wanted, all I ever wanted was to love and be loved
To need selflessly and to be needed wholly and fully.
To understand completion, to know that
My spirit is guiding me in the darkness of the void
When I am lost on my way.
To feel that I am not simply waking up
And drifting to slumber
Each day and every night
To simply repeat this monotonous melody
Over and over again
With no hope of a respite.
For the first time,
I have kissed lips
And with the parting of the two petals,
I could finally taste the sweetest nectar
That I have been deprived of for so so long.
A pomegranate cut open to reveal
The glistening rubies within.
I could touch and savor touch.
The soft pads of my fingers slowly tracing circles of
Eternity on my partner's skin
Teasing with pleasure,
Finally succumbing after anticipation.
Feeling the weight of another on me,
The load not oppressive but gratifying,
Knowing that I am forever bound to another
In body and mind.
The only thing left that I crave

That we crave

Is recognition.

More than recognition of my existence

But recognition of our existence

As one.

Just as all others have received

I beg, I implore to receive this gift too.

I ask why I am not eligible, why we are not eligible.

Why because one thread of our common tapestry

Distinguishes us as different,

Just as hair color and height differentiates all humans,

Not I but we must suffer.

Dispossessed of God's gift

And His will.

WEIGHTLESS

There was a lake behind the gardens
Of our summer home in Montauk.
And there was an ancient weeping willow at its edge
Her long branches gently caressing the still water
Always protecting the water from intrusion,
From disruption.
But that didn't stop my dad from hanging a strong rope
From the highest branch
So James and I could spend hours on end
Swinging from the wet grass
Into the crisp water with a loud holler.
There was that initial fear,
Maybe the rope wouldn't hold our weight
Maybe the branch would break.
All was forgotten when we let go and
For that one second, we were
Weightless, like astronauts or angels.
The closest I came to seeing God outside the Church.
And then, the icy relief of the water, reminding us of the
Powerful sensation of being alive.
I will swing again soon.
But this time,
There will not be anything to catch me.

A PERFECT WAY TO START THE DAY

Breakfast used to be my favorite part of the day. I was one of those people who would experiment with eggs Benedict, quiche Lorraine, maybe a stack of decadent whole-wheat almond pancakes. One slice of baguette bought that morning (at the same place where I buy The Post) spread with jam (my favorite: apricots). A bowl of mixed berries, melon, perhaps some pomegranate seeds if they have them in the store. And finally, standing guard over my colorful plate like two steadfast soldiers: the demitasse of espresso and a larger glass of freshly squeezed orange juice. The perfect way to start any day.

It was hard but I've gotten used to the grey grits and mushy pile of scrambled eggs that adorn my undistinguished plate. I take a long time to chew, contemplating the textures of which there are only two gradations: lumpy and hard. I drink my orange juice that comes out of a carton and plan what books I am going to take out of the library until the apish brute next to me knocks the juice out of my hands, spilling it all over my freshly laundered uniform, and swipes my bread and preserves.

Sartre was right. Hell is other people.

THE ORCHESTRA

I count myself lucky.
I've played violin since the age of nine.
Added piano six months later.
The music is within me.
My heart the eternal metronome.
My soul the genius composer.

At first thought,
This place doesn't exactly inspire creativity.

The walls are bare. No scenes of nature
For a new interpretation of Vivaldi's *Four Seasons*.
If there were a window, I would only see dead grass
Instead of the whispering of the tide.
Heavy footsteps don't have any tone to them.
And shouting matches are not conducive
To symphonic rhapsodies.

But…my cellie is a reader and when
He turns the pages of the latest bestseller,
The worn paper crinkles,
Revealing the mystery of the next page.

The toilet runs constantly
Like the tumbling rhythm of a stream.

And…there it is…today's punching contest seems like
The reliable thumps of the timpani.

Perhaps I have things to work with after all.

ANXIOUSLY AWAITED

I have spent years in school,
Endless studying for a license I would earn
At the end of a long tunnel.
I spent five years courting the woman who would
Become my wife,
But in reality, it was much more if you count the hours
That I lay awake dreaming about her.
And I experienced the bliss of fatherhood
In my late thirties,
Finally making the transition from boy to man
In my middle age.
I'm a patient man.

I'm a patient man but not when it comes to this.
When it comes to a sound.
A flicker on a screen.
Seconds are silently converted into lifetimes as
He or she lies still on the bed
Quietly, marked by the absence of life,
The propulsion of blood
The lack of oxygen.
Accompanied by a monotone beep that shortens my life
Every second that it continues.
It mocks me.
Renders me powerless in the face of all my education.
All my love.

My own life.

All I can do is struggle and wait for the reliable beeps

The rosy hue returning to their faces

The end of my torture.

THE STAIRS THAT STARE

It used to be easy.
In the most graceful of movements, I would lift my shoe
Up and place it on the stair.
Confident in my balance
Assured of my abilities
I doubted myself in differential equations class
But not when it came to stairs.

Perhaps I spoke too soon.
Now you, ornately decorated staircase
With looping whorls of cast-iron and polished parquet,
I have deemed thee my enemy
Your beautiful façade is deceptive
For you are unforgiving.

People tell me I should try again
No matter that I have not done this exercise in months!
They look at me with expectation, wide eyes dilating
With hope, with excitement.
But it is I who inhabits this body
I know my limits.

They are relentless
So I try again.
Hmmmm, for some reason it seems easier this time

Except the floor mocks me with its rich pallor.
I hide mine with copious amounts of blush
That makes me look like a clown.

Is it just like riding a bike?
Let's find out.
One shoe up.
A little shaky.
There we go.
Another one up
But I lose my stability in that brief moment of time
When I reach for the banister.

It was hard.
A little scary since Mom wasn't there (she was at work).
Between you and me, she would kill me if she knew I
Tried this myself.
But I did it.
The rest are higher.
More steep.
A lot more difficult, a lot more endurance required.
I'll try.
I've always wanted to climb Mount Everest.

ABOUT THE AUTHOR

SHIRIN KARIMI is an award-winning author and honors student who bridged two seemingly disparate branches of knowledge in her undergraduate years at American University, pursuing a career in medicine while fulfilling her creative side with a major in Literature. She is the recipient of the Victor Hassine Memorial Scholarship, the Outstanding Honors Junior Award, an Honorable Mention for the Best Natural Sciences Poster by a Junior or Senior at the Robyn Rafferty Mathias Student Research Conference for her presentation on antimicrobial synthesis, and BleakHouse Publishing's Tacenda Literary Short Story Award for her story, "The Desperation Diaries," published as the lead story in *BleakHouse Review*. Karimi combines her volunteer work at the Pediatric Oncology clinic of the Lombardi Cancer Center of Georgetown University Hospital with her roles as Consulting Editor of BleakHouse Publishing, Co-Editor of *Catalyst* Science Magazine, and Editor-in-Chief and contributor to *Tacenda Literary Magazine*. Her passion for writing and editing led her to be chosen as a copy-editor for two books, *A Zoo Near You* (BleakHouse Publishing, 2010) and *Miller's Revenge* (Brown Paper Publishing, 2010).

ABOUT THE DESIGNERS

LIZ CALKA is an award-winning photographer and designer recently graduated from American University. She is the Art Director of BleakHouse Publishing. Calka has always been drawn to the arts and strongly believes in the power of visuals. She has designed many book and magazine covers for BleakHouse Publishing, and she also created the BleakHouse Publishing website.

SONIA TABRIZ is a merit scholar and J.D. candidate at The George Washington University Law School. She is the Managing Editor of BleakHouse Publishing and has designed the text for several books and journals. Tabriz is best known for her award-winning works of fiction, including poetry and short stories, as well as her legal commentaries. She also co-edited and contributed to *Lethal Rejection: Stories on Crime and Punishment* (Carolina Academic Press, 2009) and *Life Without Parole: Living and Dying in Prison Today* (Oxford University Press 5th Ed., 2011).

www.ingramcontent.com/pod-product-compliance
Lightning Source LLC
Chambersburg PA
CBHW071838290426
44109CB00017B/1857